A Guide to Anti-Inflammatory Diet Recipes 2021

The Ultimate Anti-Inflammatory Guide to Fat-Proof Your Body and Restore Your Health

Joy Sanford

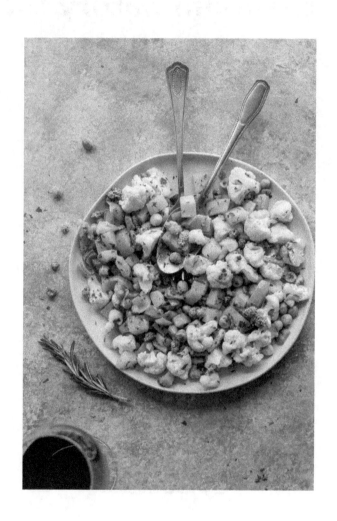

Table of Contents

Introduction

Most of the widely consumed diets incorporate anti-inflammation diet principles. In particular, the Mediterranean diet has whole grains, fish, and fats that are beneficial for the heart. Studies suggest that this diet can help lower the effects of cardiovascular system inflammation due to diet. Taking an anti-inflammatory diet is can be a complementary therapy for most conditions that are aggravated by chronic inflammation.

An anti-inflammation diet entails eating only particular kinds of food and avoiding others to lower the symptoms of chronic inflammatory diseases. It is one of the recommended measures that an individual can take to reduce or prevent inflammation induced by diet.

Expectedly, an anti-inflammatory diet involves nutrient-dense plant foods and minimizing or avoiding processed meats and foods. The goal of an anti-inflammation diet is to minimize inflammatory responses. The diet entails substituting refined foods with whole and nutrient-laden foods. Predictably, an anti-inflammation diet will contain more amounts of antioxidants that are reactive molecules in food and help reduce the number of free radicals. The free radicals are molecules in the human body that may harm cells and enhance the risk of certain diseases.

In particular, an anti-inflammation diet can help with the following diseases/conditions:

- Diabetes

Focusing exclusively on type 2 diabetes arises when the body fails to properly utilize insulin leading to higher than normal blood sugar levels. The condition of more sugar levels in the blood than normal is also known as hyperglycemia. It is also called insulin resistance. At the beginning of type 2 diabetes, the pancreas tries to make more insulin but fails to catch up with the rising blood sugar levels.

- Inflammatory bowel disease

Inflammatory bowel disease is a common gastrointestinal disorder that affects the large intestine. The symptoms of inflammatory bowel disease include abdominal pain, cramping, bloating, constipation, and diarrhea. It is a chronic condition, and it has to be managed in the long-term. Dietary measures are necessary to prevent diet-induced bloating, abdominal pain, diarrhea, and constipation. However, only a small percentage of individuals with inflammatory bowel disease will have extreme symptoms manifestation.

- Obesity

Medically, obesity refers to a complex disorder involving excessive amounts of body fat. Expectedly, obesity increases the risk of heart diseases as well as other health problems. Fortunately, modest weight loss can help halt and reverse the effects of obesity. Dietary adjustments can help address the causes of obesity, and the anti-inflammatory diet is inherently a healthy diet.

- Heart disease

Cardiovascular diseases can be triggered by diet, and diet can is used to manage several heart diseases. Food-related factors that increase the risk of heart diseases include obesity and high blood pressure. The type of fat eaten can also worsen or lesser risk of developing heart disease. In particular, cholesterol, saturated and trans fats are thought to increase heart attack rates. Most obese individuals also tend to have high-fat diets.

- Metabolic syndrome

Medically, metabolic syndrome refers to a group of factors that manifest together, leading to an increase in the risk of developing other inflammatory conditions. Some of these conditions include high blood pressure, excess body fat, especially around the waist, abnormal cholesterol, and high blood sugar levels. Having any or all of these conditions signifies that you are at a higher risk of developing a chronic condition. Most of these conditions are also associated with consuming an inflammation diet.

- Hashimoto's disease

Hashimoto's disease is an autoimmune disorder in which the body attacks its own tissues and, in particular, the thyroid organ. The result of unmanaged Hashimoto's disease is hypothyroidism implying that the body will not make adequate hormones. The thyroid gland makes hormones that control body metabolism, which includes heart rate and calories utilization. Unchecked Hashimoto's disease will also result in difficulties in swallowing when goiter manifests. Diet adjustments can be used to help manage the disease along with medications.

- Lupus

Lupus is another autoimmune disease that occurs when the body attacks its own organs and tissues. The inflammation occasioned by unmanaged lupus will affect other parts of the body. For instance, inflammation triggered by lupus will affect the heart, lungs, kidneys, and skin, including the brain and blood cells. The common symptoms of lupus are fever, fatigue, chest pain, dry eyes, and butterfly-shaped rash. Diet can be used to minimize the worsening of inflammation by adhering to the anti-inflammatory diet.

The other benefit of taking an anti-inflammation diet is that it can help lower the risk of select cancers such as colorectal cancer.

Sesame Wings with Cauliflower

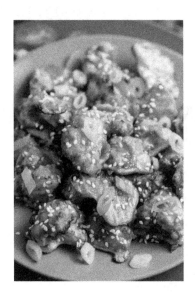

Preparation Time: 5 minutes

Cooking Time: 30 minutes

Servings: 4

Ingredients:

- 2 ½ tablespoons soy sauce

- 2 tablespoons sesame oil

- 1 ½ teaspoons balsamic vinegar

- 1 teaspoon minced garlic

- 1 teaspoon grated ginger
- Salt
- 1-pound chicken wing, the wings itself
- 2 cups cauliflower florets

Directions:

1. In a freezer bag, mix the soy sauce, sesame oil, balsamic vinegar, garlic, ginger, and salt, then add the chicken wings.
2. Coat flip, then chill for 2 to 3 hours.
3. Preheat the oven to 400 F and line a foil-based baking sheet.
4. Spread the wings along with the cauliflower onto the baking sheet.
5. Bake for 35 minutes, then sprinkle on to serve with sesame seeds.

Nutrition: Calories: 400 Fats: 15 Protein: 5 Carbohydrates: 3

Fried Coconut Shrimp with Asparagus

Preparation Time: 15 minutes

Cooking Time: 10 minutes

Servings: 6

Ingredients:

- 1 ½ cups shredded unsweetened coconut
- 2 large eggs
- Salt and pepper
- 1 ½ pounds large shrimp, peeled and deveined
- ½ cup canned coconut milk
- 1-pound asparagus, cut into 2-inch pieces

Directions:

1. Pour the coconut onto a shallow platter.
2. Beat the eggs in a bowl with a little salt and pepper.
3. Dip the shrimp into the egg first, then dredge with coconut.

4. Heat up coconut oil over medium-high heat in a large skillet.

5. Add the shrimp and fry over each side for 1 to 2 minutes until browned.

6. Remove the paper towels from the shrimp and heat the skillet again.

7. Remove the asparagus and sauté to tender-crisp with salt and pepper, then serve with the shrimp.

Nutrition: Calories: 535 Fats: 38 Protein: 16 Carbohydrates: 3

Coconut Chicken Curry with Cauliflower Rice

Preparation Time: 15 minutes

Cooking Time: 30 minutes

Servings: 6

Ingredients:

- 1 tablespoon olive oil
- 1 medium yellow onion, chopped
- 1 ½ pounds boneless chicken thighs, chopped
- Salt and pepper
- 1 (14-ounce) can coconut milk
- 1 tablespoon curry powder
- 1 ¼ teaspoon ground turmeric
- 3 cups riced cauliflower

Directions:

1. Heat the oil over medium heat, in a large skillet.
2. Add the onions, and cook for about 5 minutes, until translucent.

3. Stir in the chicken and season with salt and pepper-cook for 6 to 8 minutes, stirring frequently until all sides are browned.

4. Pour the coconut milk into the pan, then whisk in the curry and turmeric powder.

5. Simmer until hot and bubbling, for 15 to 20 minutes.

6. Meanwhile, steam the cauliflower rice until tender with a few tablespoons of water.

7. Serve the cauliflower rice over the curry.

Nutrition: Calories: 430 Fats: 29 Protein: 9 Carbohydrates: 3

Pumpkin Spiced Almonds

Preparation Time: 5 minutes

Cooking Time: 25 minutes

Servings: 4

Ingredients:

- 1 tablespoon olive oil
- 1 ¼ teaspoon pumpkin pie spice
- Pinch salt
- 1 cup whole almonds, raw

Direction:

- Preheat the oven to 300 ° F, and line a parchment baking sheet.
- In a mixing bowl, whisk together the olive oil, pumpkin pie spice, and salt.
- Toss in the almonds until coated evenly, then scatter onto the baking sheet.
- Bake and place in an airtight container for 25 minutes then cool down completely.

Nutrition: Calories: 170 Fats: 15 Protein: 5 Carbohydrates: 3

Tzatziki Dip with Cauliflower

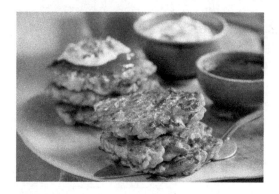

Preparation Time: 10 minutes

Cooking Time: 0 minutes

Servings: 6

Ingredients:

1. ½ (8-ounce) package cream cheese, softened
2. 1 cup sour cream
3. 1 tablespoon ranch seasoning
4. 1 English cucumber, diced
5. 2 tablespoons chopped chives
6. 2 cups cauliflower florets

Directions:

1. Use an electric mixer to pound the cream cheese until smooth.
2. Stir in the sour cream and ranch seasoning, beat until smooth.
3. Fold in the cucumbers and chives, then chill with cauliflower florets for dipping before serving.

Nutrition: Calories: 125 Fats: 10 Protein: 5 Carbohydrates: 3

Classic Guacamole Dip

Preparation Time: 15 minutes

Cooking Time: 0 minutes

Servings: 4

Ingredients:

- 2 mediums avocado, pitted
- 1 small yellow onion, diced
- 1 small tomato, diced
- ¼ cup fresh chopped cilantro
- 1 tablespoon fresh lime juice
- 1 jalapeno, seeded and minced
- 1 clove garlic, minced
- Salt
- Sliced veggies to serve

Directions:

- Mash avocado flesh into a bowl.
- Stir the onion, tomato, cilantro, lime juice, garlic, and jalapeno in a bowl
- Season lightly with salt and spoon into a bowl – serve with sliced veggies.

Nutrition: Calories: 225 Fats: 20 Protein: 12
Carbohydrates: 3

Creamy Queso Dip

Preparation Time: 15 minutes

Cooking Time: 5 minutes

Servings: 8

Ingredients:

1. 4 ounces chorizo, crumbled

2. 1 clove garlic, minced

3. ¼ cup heavy cream

4. 6 ounces shredded white cheddar cheese

5. 2 ounces shredded pepper jack cheese

6. ¼ teaspoon xanthan gum

7. Pinch salt

8. 1 jalapeno, seeded and minced

9. 1 small tomato, diced

Directions:

1. Cook the chorizo in a skillet until browned evenly, then scatter in a dish.

2. At medium-low heat, pressure the skillet and add the garlic–cook for 30 seconds.

3. Stir in the heavy cream, then add the cheese a little at a time, stirring frequently until it melts.

4. Sprinkle with salt and xanthan gum, then mix well, and cook until thickened.

5. Add the tomato and jalapeno, then serve, dipping with vegetables.

Nutrition: Calories: 195 Fats: 16 Protein: 12 Carbohydrates: 1

Herb Butter Scallops

Preparation Time: 10 minutes

Cooking Time: 10 minutes

Servings: 3

Ingredients:

- 1 pound sea scallops, cleaned
- Freshly ground black pepper
- 8 tablespoons butter, divided
- 2 teaspoons minced garlic
- Juice of 1 lemon
- 2 teaspoons chopped fresh basil
- 1 teaspoon chopped fresh thyme

Directions:

1. Pat the scallops dry with paper towels and season them lightly with pepper.
2. Place a large skillet over medium heat and add 2 tablespoons of butter.
3. Arrange the scallops in the skillet, evenly spaced but not too close together, and sear

each side until they are golden brown, about 2½ minutes per side.

4. Remove the scallops to a plate and set aside.

5. Add the remaining 6 tablespoons of butter to the skillet and sauté the garlic until translucent, about 3 minutes.

6. Stir in the lemon juice, basil, and thyme and return the scallops to the skillet, turning to coat them in the sauce.

7. Serve immediately.

Nutrition:

Calories: 306 Fat: 24g Protein: 19g carbohydrates: 4g Fiber: 0g

Dinner

Pan-Seared Halibut with Citrus Butter Sauce

Preparation Time: 10 minutes

Cooking Time: 15 minutes

Servings: 3

Ingredients:

- 4 (5-ounce) halibut fillets, each about 1 inch thick
- Sea salt
- Freshly ground black pepper
- ¼ cup butter
- 2 teaspoons minced garlic
- 1 shallot, minced
- 3 tablespoons dry white wine
- 1 tablespoon freshly squeezed lemon juice
- 1 tablespoon freshly squeezed orange juice
- 2 teaspoons chopped fresh parsley

- 2 tablespoons olive oil

Directions:

1. Pat the fish dry with paper towels and then lightly season the fillets with salt and pepper. Set aside on a paper towel–lined plate.

2. Place a small saucepan over medium heat and melt the butter.

3. Sauté the garlic and shallot until tender, about 3 minutes.

4. Whisk in the white wine, lemon juice, and orange juice and bring the sauce to a simmer, cooking until it thickens slightly, about 2 minutes.

5. Remove the sauce from the heat and stir in the parsley; set aside.

6. Place a large skillet over medium-high heat and add the olive oil.

7. Panfry the fish until lightly browned and just cooked through, turning them over once, about 10 minutes in total.

8. Serve the fish immediately with a spoonful of sauce for each.

Nutrition: Calories: 319 Fat: 26g Protein: 22g Carbohydrates: 2g Fiber: 0g

Sole Asiago

Preparation Time: 10 minutes

Cooking Time: 8 minutes

Servings: 4

Ingredients:

- 4 (4-ounce) sole fillets
- ¾ cup ground almonds
- ¼ cup Asiago cheese
- 2 eggs, beaten
- 2½ tablespoons melted coconut oil

Directions:

1. Preheat the oven to 350°F. Line a baking sheet with parchment paper and set aside.
2. Pat the fish dry with paper towels.
3. Stir together the ground almonds and cheese in a small bowl.
4. Place the bowl with the beaten eggs in it next to the almond mixture.
5. Dredge a sole fillet in the beaten egg and then press the fish into the almond mixture

so it is completely coated. Place on the baking sheet and repeat until all the fillets are breaded.

6. Brush both sides of each piece of fish with the coconut oil.
7. Bake the sole until it is cooked through, about 8 minutes in total.
8. Serve immediately.

Nutrition: Calories: 406 Fat: 31g Protein: 29g carbohydrates: 6g Fiber: 3g

Cheesy Garlic Salmon

Preparation Time: 15 minutes

Cooking Time: 12 minutes

Servings: 4

Ingredients:

- ½ cup Asiago cheese
- 2 tablespoons freshly squeezed lemon juice
- 2 tablespoons butter, at room temperature
- 2 teaspoons minced garlic
- 1 teaspoon chopped fresh basil
- 1 teaspoon chopped fresh oregano
- 4 (5-ounce) salmon fillets
- 1 tablespoon olive oil

Directions:

1. Preheat the oven to 350°F. Line a baking sheet with parchment paper and set aside.
2. In a small bowl, stir together the Asiago cheese, lemon juice, butter, garlic, basil, and oregano.

3. Pat the salmon dry with paper towels and place the fillets on the baking sheet skin-side down. Divide the topping evenly between the fillets and spread it across the fish using a knife or the back of a spoon.

4. Drizzle the fish with the olive oil and bake until the topping is golden and the fish is just cooked through, about 12 minutes.

5. Serve.

Nutrition: Calories: 357 Fat: 28g Protein: 24g Carbohydrates: 2g Fiber: 0g

Stuffed Chicken Breasts

Preparation Time: 30 minutes

Cooking Time: 30 minutes

Servings: 4

Ingredients:

- 1 tablespoon butter
- ¼ cup chopped sweet onion
- ½ cup goat cheese, at room temperature
- ¼ cup Kalamata olives, chopped
- ¼ cup chopped roasted red pepper
- 2 tablespoons chopped fresh basil
- 4 (5-ounce) chicken breasts, skin-on
- 2 tablespoons extra-virgin olive oil

Directions:

1. Preheat the oven to 400°F.
2. In a small skillet over medium heat, melt the butter and add the onion. Sauté until tender, about 3 minutes.
3. Transfer the onion to a medium bowl and add the cheese, olives, red pepper, and

basil. Stir until well blended, then refrigerate for about 30 minutes.

4. Cut horizontal pockets into each chicken breast, and stuff them evenly with the filling. Secure the two sides of each breast with toothpicks.

5. Place a large ovenproof skillet over medium-high heat and add the olive oil.

6. Brown the chicken on both sides, about 10 minutes in total.

7. Place the skillet in the oven and roast until the chicken is just cooked through, about 15 minutes. Remove the toothpicks and serve.

Nutrition: Calories: 389 Fat: 30g Protein: 25g Carbohydrates: 3g Fiber: 0g

Spicy Pork Chops

Preparation Time: 4 hours and 10 minutes

Cooking Time: 15 minutes

Servings: 2

Ingredients:

- ¼ cup lime juice 2 pork rib chops
- 1/2 tablespoon coconut oil, melted
- 1/2 garlic cloves, peeled and minced
- 1/2 tablespoon chili powder
- 1/2 teaspoon ground cinnamon
- 1 teaspoon cumin
- Salt and pepper to taste
- 1/4 teaspoon hot pepper sauce
- Mango, sliced

Directions:

1. Take a bowl and mix in lime juice, oil, garlic, cumin, cinnamon, chili powder, salt, pepper, hot pepper sauce. Whisk well.
2. Add pork chops and toss. Keep it on the side, and let it refrigerate for 4 hours.

3. Preheat your grill to medium and transfer pork chops to the preheated grill. Grill for 7 minutes, flip and cook for 7 minutes more.

4. Divide between serving platters and serve with mango slices. Enjoy!

Nutrition: Calories: 200 | Fat: 8g | Carbohydrates: 3g | Protein: 26g | Fiber: 1g | Net Carbohydrates: 2g

Almond Breaded Chicken Goodness

Preparation Time: 15 minutes

Cooking Time: 15 minutes

Servings: 2

Ingredients:

- 2 large chicken breast, boneless and skinless
- 1/3 cup lemon juice
- 1½ cups seasoned almond meal
- 2 tablespoons coconut oil
- Lemon pepper, to taste
- Parsley for decoration

Directions:

1. Slice Hicken breast in half.
2. Pound out each half until a ¼ inch thick.
3. Put a pan over medium heat, add oil and heat it.
4. Dip each chicken breast slice into lemon juice and let it sit for 2 minutes.

5. Turnover and let the other side sit for 2 minutes as well.

6. Transfer to almond meal and coat both sides.

7. Add coated chicken to the oil and fry for 4 minutes per side, making sure to sprinkle lemon pepper liberally.

8. Transfer to a paper-lined sheet and repeat until all chicken is fried.

9. Garnish with parsley and enjoy.

Nutrition: Calories: 325 | Fat: 24g | Carbohydrates: 3g | Protein: 16g | Fiber: 1g | Net Carbohydrates: 1g

Garlic Lamb Chops

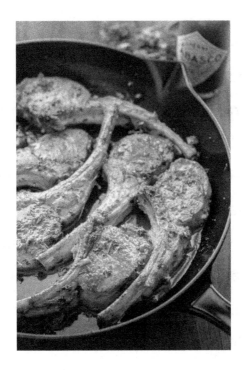

Preparation Time: 35 minutes

Cooking Time: 5 minutes

Servings: 2

Ingredients:

- ¼ cup olive oil

- ¼ cup mint, fresh and chopped

- 8 lamb rib chops

- 1 tablespoon garlic, minced
- 1 tablespoon rosemary, fresh and chopped

Directions:

1. Add rosemary, garlic, mint, olive oil into a bowl and mix well.
2. Keep a tablespoon of the mixture on the side for later use.
3. Toss lamb chops into the marinade, letting them marinate for 30 minutes.
4. Preheat the cast-iron skillet over medium-high heat.
5. Add lamb and cook for 2 minutes per side for medium-rare.
6. Let the lamb rest for a few minutes and drizzle the remaining marinade.
7. Serve and enjoy!

Nutrition: Calories: 566 | Fat: 40g | Carbohydrates: 2g | Protein: 47g | Fiber: 1g | Net Carbohydrates: 1g

Mushroom Pork Chops

Preparation Time: 10 minutes

Cooking Time: 40 minutes

Servings: 2

Ingredients:

- 8 ounces mushrooms, sliced
- 1 teaspoon garlic
- 1 onion, peeled and chopped
- 1 cup keto-friendly mayonnaise
- 3 pork chops, boneless
- 1 teaspoon ground nutmeg
- 1 tablespoon balsamic vinegar
- ½ cup of coconut oil

Directions:

1. Take a pan and place it over medium heat. Add oil and let it heat up. Add mushrooms, onions, and stir. Cook for 4 minutes.

2. Add pork chops, season with nutmeg, garlic powder, and brown both sides. Transfer the pan in the oven and bake for 30 minutes at

350 degrees F. Transfer pork chops to plates and keeps it warm.

3. Take a pan and place it over medium heat. Add vinegar, mayonnaise over the mushroom mixture, and stir for a few minutes.

4. Drizzle sauce over pork chops

5. Enjoy!

Nutrition: Calories: 600 | Fat: 10g | Carbohydrates: 8g | Protein: 30g | Fiber: 2g | Net Carbohydrates: 5g

Mediterranean Pork

Preparation Time: 10 minutes

Cooking Time: 35 minutes

Servings: 2

Ingredients:

- 2 pork chops, bone-in
- Salt and pepper, to taste
- 1/2 teaspoon dried rosemary
- 1 garlic clove, peeled and minced

Directions:

1. Season pork chops with salt and pepper. Place in a roasting pan. Add rosemary, garlic in the pan.

2. Preheat your oven to 425 degrees F. Bake for 10 minutes. Lower heat to 350 degrees F. Roast for 25 minutes more. Slice pork and divide on plates.

3. Drizzle pan juice all over. Serve and enjoy!

Nutrition: Calories: 165 | Fat: 2g | Carbohydrates: 2g | Protein: 26g | Fiber: 1g | Net Carbohydrates: 1g

Brie-Packed Smoked Salmon

Preparation Time: 4 minutes

Cooking Time: 0 minutes

Servings: 4

Ingredients:

- 4 ounce Brie round
- 1 tablespoon fresh dill
- 1 tablespoon lemon juice
- 2-ounce smoked salmon

Directions:

1. Slice Brie in half lengthwise.
2. Spread salmon, dill, and lemon juice over the Brie cheese.
3. Place the other half on top.
4. Serve with Celery sticks/ cauliflower bites.
5. Enjoy!

Nutrition: Calories: 241 | Fat: 19g | Net Carbohydrates: 0g | Protein: 18g | Fiber: 2g | Carbohydrates: 3g

Blackened Tilapia

Preparation Time: 9 minutes

Cooking Time: 9 minutes

Servings: 2

Ingredients:

- 1 cup cauliflower, chopped
- 1 teaspoon red pepper flakes
- 1 tablespoon Italian seasoning
- 1 tablespoon garlic, minced
- 6 ounce tilapia
- 1 cup English cucumber, chopped with peel
- 2 tablespoon olive oil
- 1 sprig dill, chopped
- 1 teaspoon stevia
- 3 tablespoon lime juice
- 2 tablespoon Cajun blackened seasoning

Directions:

1. Take a bowl and add the seasoning
   ingredients (except Cajun). Add a
   tablespoon of oil and whip. Pour dressing

over cauliflower and cucumber. Brush the fish with olive oil on both sides.

2. Take a skillet and grease it well with 1 tablespoon of olive oil. Press Cajun seasoning on both sides of the fish.

3. Cook fish for 3 minutes per side. Serve with vegetables and enjoy!

Nutrition: Calories: 530 | Fat: 33g | Net Carbohydrates: 4g | Protein: 32g | Fiber: 2g | Carbohydrates: 2g

Salsa Chicken Bites

Preparation Time: 4 minutes

Cooking Time: 14 minutes

Servings: 2

Ingredients:

- 2 chicken rest
- 1 cup of salsa
- 1 taco seasoning mix
- 1 cup plain Greek yogurt
- ½ cup cheddar cheese, cubed

Directions:

1. Take a skillet and place it over medium heat.
2. Add chicken breast, a ½ cup of salsa, and taco seasoning.
3. Mix well and cook for 12-15 minutes until the chicken is done.
4. Take the chicken out and cube them.
5. Place the cubes on toothpick and top with cheddar.

6. Place yogurt and remaining salsa in cups and use them as dips.

7. Serve and Enjoy!

Nutrition: Calories: 359 | Fat: 14g | Net Carbohydrates: 14g | Protein: 43g | Fiber: 3g | Carbohydrates: 17g

Tomato & Tuna Balls

Preparation Time: 25 minutes

Cooking Time: 0

Servings: 2

Ingredients:

- 8 tomatoes, medium
- 1 tablespoon of capers
- 2 – 3-ounce cans tuna, drained
- 10 Kalamata olives, pitted and minced
- 2 tablespoon parsley
- 1 tablespoon olive oil
- ½ teaspoon thyme
- Salt, to taste
- pepper, as needed

Directions:

1. Line a cookie pan with a paper towel and scoop guts out from the tomatoes.
2. Keep the tomato shells on the side.
3. Take a bowl and mix olives, tuna, thyme, parsley, pepper in a bowl and mix.

4. Add oil and mix.

5. Fill the tomato shells with tuna mix.

6. Enjoy!

Nutrition: Calories: 169 | Fat: 10g | Net Carbohydrates: 5g | Protein: 13g | Fiber: 5g | Carbohydrates: 10g

Fennel & Figs Lamb

Preparation Time: 10 minutes

Cooking Time: 40 minutes

Servings: 2

Ingredients:

- 6 ounces lamb racks
- 1 fennel bulbs, sliced
- Salt
- pepper, to taste
- 1 tablespoon olive oil
- 2 figs, cut in half
- 1/8 cup apple cider vinegar
- 1/2 tablespoon swerve

Directions:

1. Take a bowl and add fennel, figs, vinegar, swerve, oil, and toss. Transfer to baking dish. Season with salt and pepper.
2. Bake it for 15 minutes at 400 degrees F.
3. Season lamb with salt, pepper, and transfer to a heated pan over medium-high heat.

Cook for a few minutes. Add lamb to the
baking dish with fennel and bake for 20
minutes. Divide between plates and serve.
Enjoy!

Nutrition: Calories: 230 | Fat: 3g | Carbohydrates:
5g | Protein: 10g | Fiber: 2g | Net Carbohydrates:
3g

Tamari Steak Salad

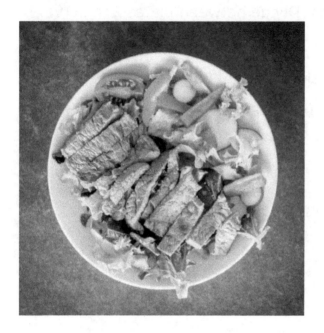

Preparation Time: 15 minutes

Cooking Time: 10 minutes

Servings: 2

Ingredients:

- 1 large bunches salad greens
- 4 ounces beef steak
- ½ red bell pepper, diced
- 4 cherry tomatoes, cut into halves

- 2 radishes, sliced

- 2 tablespoons olive oil

- ¼ tablespoon fresh lemon juice

- 1-ounce gluten-free tamari sauce

- Salt as needed

Directions:

1. Marinate steak in tamari sauce.

2. Make the salad by adding bell pepper, tomatoes, radishes, salad green, oil, salt, and lemon juice to a bowl and toss them well.

3. Grill the steak to your desired doneness and transfer steak on top of the salad platter.

4. Let it sit for 1 minute and cut it crosswise.

5. Serve and enjoy!

Nutrition: Calories: 500 | Fat: 37g | Carbohydrates: 4g | Protein: 33g | Fiber: 2g | Net Carbohydrates: 2g

Blackened Chicken

Preparation Time: 10 minutes

Cooking Time: 10 minutes

Servings: 2

Ingredients:

- 1/4 teaspoon paprika
- 1/8 teaspoon salt
- ¼ teaspoon cayenne pepper
- ¼ teaspoon ground cumin
- ¼ teaspoon dried thyme
- 1/8 teaspoon ground white pepper
- 1/8 teaspoon onion powder
- 1 chicken breast, boneless and skinless

Directions:

- Preheat your oven to 350 degrees Fahrenheit. Grease baking sheet. Take a cast-iron skillet and place it over high heat.
- Add oil and heat it for 5 minutes until smoking hot.

- Take a small bowl and mix salt, paprika, cumin, white pepper, cayenne, thyme, onion powder. Oil the chicken breast on both sides and coat the breast with the spice mix.
- Transfer to your hot pan and cook for 1 minute per side.
- Transfer to your prepared baking sheet and bake for 5 minutes.
- Serve and enjoy!

Nutrition: Calories: 136 | Fat: 3g | Carbohydrates: 2g | Protein: 24g | Fiber: 1g | Net Carbohydrates: 1g

Mediterranean Mushroom Olive Steak

Preparation Time: 10 minutes

Cooking Time: 14 minutes

Servings: 2

Ingredients:

- 1/2 pound boneless beef sirloin steak, ¾ inch thick, cut into 4 pieces
- 1/2 large red onion, chopped
- 1/2 cup mushrooms
- 2 garlic cloves, thinly sliced
- 2 tablespoons olive oil
- 1/4 cup green olives, coarsely chopped
- 1/2 cup parsley leaves, finely cut

Directions:

1. Take a large-sized skillet and place it over medium-high heat.
2. Add oil and let it heat up. Add beef and cook until both sides are browned, remove beef

and drain fat. Add the rest of the oil to the skillet and heat it.

3. Add onions, garlic, and cook for 2-3 minutes. Stir well.

4. Add mushrooms olives and cook until mushrooms are thoroughly done. Return beef to skillet and lower heat to medium.

5. Cook for 3-4 minutes (covered). Stir in parsley.

6. Serve and enjoy!

Nutrition: Calories: 386 | Fat: 30g | Carbohydrates: 11g | Protein: 21g | Fiber: 5g | Net Carbohydrates: 6g

Buttery Scallops

Preparation Time: 10 minutes

Cooking Time: 10 minutes

Servings: 6

Ingredients:

- 2 pounds sea scallops
- 3 tablespoons butter, melted
- 2 tablespoons fresh thyme, minced
- Salt and pepper, to taste

Directions:

1. Preheat your air fryer to 390 degrees F. Grease the air fryer cooking basket with butter.
2. Take a bowl, mix in all of the remaining ingredients, and toss well to coat the scallops.
3. Transfer scallops to air fryer-cooking basket and cook for 5 minutes.
4. Repeat if any ingredients are left, serve, and enjoy!

Nutrition: Calories: 186, Total Fat: 24g, Total Carbs: 4g, Fiber: 1g, Net Carbs: 2g, Protein: 20g

Brussels sprouts and Garlic Aioli

Preparation Time: 15 minutes

Cooking Time: 10 minutes

Servings: 4

Ingredients:

1 pound Brussels sprouts, trimmed and excess leaves removed

Salt and pepper, to taste

1½ tablespoons olive oil

2 teaspoons lemon juice

1 teaspoon powdered chili

3 garlic cloves

¾ cup whole egg, keto-friendly mayonnaise

2 cups of water

Directions:

Take a skillet and place it over medium heat.

Add garlic cloves (with peel) and roast until brown and fragrant.

Remove skillet with garlic and put a pot with water over medium heat, bring the water to a boil.

Take a knife and cut Brussels sprouts in halves lengthwise, add them to the boiling water, blanch for 3 minutes.

Drain them through a sieve and keep them on the side.

Preheat your air fryer to 350 degrees F.

Remove garlic from skillet and peel, crush them, and keep them on the side.

Add olive oil to skillet and place it over medium heat, stir in Brussels and season with salt and pepper, cook for 2 minutes.

Remove heat and transfer sprouts to your air fryer cooking basket, cook for 5 minutes. Make aioli by taking a small bowl and add mayonnaise, crushed garlic, lemon juice, powdered chili, pepper, salt, and mix.

Serve Brussels with the aioli, enjoy!

Nutrition: Calories: 42, Total Fat: 2g, Total Carbs: 3g, Fiber: 1g, Net Carbs: 2g, Protein: 5g

Broccoli Bites

Preparation Time: 15 minutes

Cooking Time: 12 minutes

Servings: 4

Ingredients:

- 2 eggs, beaten
- ¼ cup parmesan cheese, grated
- 2 cups broccoli florets
- 1½ cups cheddar cheese, grated
- Salt and pepper, to taste

Directions:

1. Add broccoli to the food processor and pulse until crumbly.
2. Mix broccoli and remaining ingredients in a large bowl.
3. Make small balls from the mixture and arrange them in a baking sheet.
4. Let it refrigerate for 30 minutes.
5. Preheat your Air Fryer to 360 degrees F.

6. Transfer balls to air fryer cooking basket and cook for 12 minutes.

7. Serve and enjoy!

Nutrition: Calories: 234, Total Fat: 17g, Total Carbs: 4g, Fiber: 1g, Net Carbs: 2g, Protein: 16g

Bacon Burger Cabbage Stir Fry

Preparation Time: 10 minutes

Cooking Time: 20 minutes

Servings: 10

Ingredients:

- Ground beef (1 lb.)
- Bacon (1 lb.) Small onion (1)
- Minced cloves of garlic (3)
- Cabbage (1 lb./1 small head)

Directions:

1. Dice the bacon and onion. Combine the beef and bacon in a wok or large skillet.
2. Prepare it until done and store it in a bowl to keep warm. Mince the onion and garlic.
3. Toss both into the hot grease. Slice and toss in the cabbage and stir-fry until wilted.
4. Blend in the meat and combine. Sprinkle with pepper and salt as desired.

Nutrition: Net Carbohydrates: 4.5 grams Protein Counts: 32 grams Total Fats: 22 grams Calories: 357

Bacon Cheeseburger

Preparation Time: 15 minutes

Cooking Time: 30 minutes

Servings: 12

Ingredients:

- Low-sodium bacon (16 oz. pkg.)
- Ground beef (3 lb.)
- Eggs (2)
- Medium chopped onion (half of 1)
- Shredded cheddar cheese (8 oz.)

Directions:

1. Fry the bacon and chop it to bits. Shred the cheese and dice the onion.
2. Combine the mixture with the beef and blend in the whisked eggs.
3. Prepare 24 burgers and grill them the way you like them.
4. You can make a double-decker since they are small.

5. If you like a bigger burger, you can make 12 burgers as a single-decker.

Nutrition: Net Carbohydrates: 0.8 grams Protein Counts: 27 grams Total Fats: 41 grams Calories: 489

Cauliflower Mac & Cheese

Preparation Time: 15 minutes

Cooking Time: 20 minutes

Servings: 4

Ingredients:

- Cauliflower (1 head)

- Butter (3 tbsp.)

- Unsweetened almond milk (.25 cup)

- Heavy cream (.25 cup)

- Cheddar cheese (1 cup)

Directions:

1. Use a sharp knife to slice the cauliflower into small florets. Shred the cheese. Prepare the oven to reach 450º Fahrenheit. Cover a baking pan with a layer of parchment baking paper or foil.

2. Add two tablespoons of the butter to a pan and melt. Add the florets, butter, salt, and pepper together. Place the cauliflower on the baking pan and roast 10 to 15 minutes.

3. Warm up the rest of the butter, milk, heavy cream, and cheese in the microwave or double boiler. Pour the cheese over the cauliflower and serve.

Nutrition: Net Carbohydrates: 7 grams Protein Counts: 11 grams Total Fats: 23 grams Calories: 294 grams

Mushroom & Cauliflower Risotto

Preparation Time: 5 minutes

Cooking Time: 10 minutes

Servings: 4

Ingredients:

- Grated head of cauliflower (1)
- Vegetable stock (1 cup)
- Chopped mushrooms (9 oz.)
- Butter (2 tbsp.)
- Coconut cream (1 cup)

Directions:

1. Pour the stock in a saucepan. Boil and set aside. Prepare a skillet with butter and saute the mushrooms until golden.
2. Grate and stir in the cauliflower and stock. Simmer and add the cream, cooking until the cauliflower is al dente. Serve.

Nutrition: Net Carbohydrates: 4 grams Protein Counts: 1 gram Total Fats: 17 grams Calories: 186

Pita Pizza

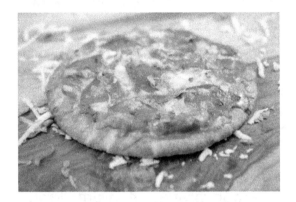

Preparation Time: 15 minutes

Cooking Time: 10 minutes

Servings: 2

Ingredients:

- Marinara sauce (.5 cup)

- Low-carb pita (1)

- Cheddar cheese (2 oz.)

- Pepperoni (14 slices)

- Roasted red peppers (1 oz.)

Directions:

1. Program the oven temperature setting to 450º Fahrenheit.

2. Slice the pita in half and place onto a foil-lined baking tray. Rub with a bit of oil and toast for one to two minutes.

3. Pour the sauce over the bread. Sprinkle using the cheese and other toppings. Bake until the cheese melts (5 min.). Cool thoroughly.

Nutrition: Net Carbohydrates: 4 grams Protein Counts: 13 grams Total Fats: 19 grams Calories: 250

Skillet Cabbage Tacos

Preparation Time: 10 minutes

Cooking Time: 15 minutes

Servings: 4

Ingredients:

- Ground beef (1 lb.)
- Salsa - ex. Pace Organic (.5 cup)
- Shredded cabbage (2 cups)
- Chili powder (2 tsp.)
- Shredded cheese (.75 cup)

Directions:

1. Brown the beef and drain the fat. Pour in the salsa, cabbage, and seasoning.
2. Cover and lower the heat. Simmer for 10 to 12 minutes using the medium heat temperature setting.
3. When the cabbage has softened, remove it from the heat and mix in the cheese.
4. Top it off using your favorite toppings, such as green onions or sour cream, and serve.

Nutrition: Net Carbohydrates: 4 gramsProtein Counts: 30 gramsTotal Fats: 21 grams Calories: 325

Taco Casserole

Preparation Time: 10 minutes

Cooking Time: 20 minutes

Servings: 8

Ingredients:

- Ground turkey or beef (1.5 to 2 lb.)
- Taco seasoning (2 tbsp.) Shredded cheddar cheese (8 oz.)
- Salsa (1 cup) Cottage cheese (16 oz.)

Directions:

1. Heat the oven to reach 400° Fahrenheit.
2. Combine the taco seasoning and ground meat in a casserole dish. Bake it for 20 minutes.
3. Combine the salsa and both kinds of cheese. Set aside for now.
4. Carefully transfer the casserole dish from the oven. Drain away the cooking juices from the meat.

5. Break the meat into small pieces and mash with a potato masher or fork.

6. Sprinkle with cheese. Bake in the oven for 15 to 20 more minutes until the top is browned.

Nutrition: Net Carbohydrates: 6 grams Protein Counts: 45 grams Total Fats: 18 grams Calories: 367

Creamy Chicken Salad

Preparation Time: 10 minutes

Cooking Time: 30 minutes

Servings: 4

Ingredients:

- Chicken Breast - 1 Lb.
- Avocado - 2
- Garlic Cloves - 2,
- Minced Lime Juice - 3 T.
- Onion - .33 C.,
- Minced Jalapeno Pepper - 1,
- Minced Salt - Dash Cilantro - 1 T.
- Pepper - Dash

Directions:

1. You will want to start this recipe off my prepping the stove to 400. As this warms up, get out your cooking sheet and line it with paper or foil.

2. Next, it is time to get out the chicken.

3. Go ahead and layer the chicken breast up with some olive oil before seasoning to your liking.

4. When the chicken is all set, you will want to line them along the surface of your cooking sheet and pop it into the oven for about twenty minutes.

5. By the end of twenty minutes, the chicken should be cooked through and can be taken out of the oven for chilling.

6. Once cool enough to handle, you will want to either dice or shred your chicken, dependent upon how you like your chicken salad.

7. Now that your chicken is all cooked, it is time to assemble your salad!

8. You can begin this process by adding everything into a bowl and mashing down the avocado.

9. Once your ingredients are mended to your liking, sprinkle some salt over the top and serve immediately.

Nutrition: Fats: 20g Carbs: 4g Proteins: 25g

Spicy Keto Chicken Wings

Preparation Time: 20 minutes

Cooking Time: 30 minutes

Servings: 4

Ingredients:

- Chicken Wings - 2 Lbs.
- Cajun Spice - 1 t.
- Smoked Paprika - 2 t.
- Turmeric - .50 t.
- Salt - Dash
- Baking Powder - 2 t.
- Pepper - Dash

Directions:

1. When you first begin the Ketogenic Diet, you may find that you won't be eating the traditional foods that may have made up a majority of your diet in the past.

2. While this is a good thing for your health, you may feel you are missing out! The good news is that there are delicious alternatives

that aren't lacking in flavor! To start this recipe, you'll want to prep the stove to 400.

3. As this heats up, you will want to take some time to dry your chicken wings with a paper towel. This will help remove any excess moisture and get you some nice, crispy wings!

4. When you are all set, take out a mixing bowl and place all of the seasonings along with the baking powder. If you feel like it, you can adjust the seasoning levels however you would like.

5. Once these are set, go ahead and throw the chicken wings in and coat evenly. If you have one, you'll want to place the wings on a wire rack that is placed over your baking tray. If not, you can just lay them across the baking sheet.

6. Now that your chicken wings are set, you are going to pop them into the stove for

thirty minutes. By the end of this time, the tops of the wings should be crispy.

7. If they are, take them out from the oven and flip them so that you can bake the other side. You will want to cook these for an additional thirty minutes.

8. Finally, take the tray from the oven and allow to cool slightly before serving up your spiced keto wings. For additional flavor, serve with any of your favorite, keto-friendly dipping sauce.

Nutrition: Fats: 7g   Carbs: 1g   Proteins: 60g

Cheesy Ham Quiche

Preparation Time: 10 minutes

Cooking Time: 30 minutes

Servings: 6

Ingredients:

- Eggs - 8
- Zucchini - 1 C.,
- Shredded heavy Cream - .50 C.
- Ham - 1 C., Diced
- Mustard - 1 t.
- Salt – Dash

Directions:

1. For this recipe, you can start off by prepping your stove to 375 and getting out a pie plate for your quiche.

2. Next, it is time to prep the zucchini. First, you will want to go ahead and shred it into small pieces.

3. Once this is complete, take a paper towel and gently squeeze out the excess moisture. This will help avoid a soggy quiche.

4. When the step from above is complete, you will want to place the zucchini into your pie plate along with the cooked ham pieces and your cheese.

5. Once these items are in place, you will want to whisk the seasonings, cream, and eggs together before pouring it over the top.

6. Now that your quiche is set, you are going to pop the dish into your stove for about forty minutes.

7. By the end of this time, the egg should be cooked through, and you will be able to insert a knife into the center and have it come out clean.

8. If the quiche is cooked to your liking, take the dish from the oven and allow it to chill slightly before slicing and serving.

Nutrition: Fats: 25g Carbs: 2g Proteins: 20g

Feta and Cauliflower Rice Stuffed Bell Peppers

Preparation Time: 10 minutes

Cooking Time: 20 minutes

Servings: 3

Ingredients:

- 1 green Bell Pepper
- 1 red Bell Pepper
- 1 yellow Bell Pepper
- ½ cup Cauliflower rice
- 1 cup Feta cheese
- 1 Onion, sliced
- 2 Tomatoes, chopped
- 1 tbsp. black Pepper
- 2-3 Garlic clove, minced
- 3 tbsp. Lemon juice
- 3-4 green Olives, chopped
- 3-4 tbsp. Olive oil
- Yogurt Sauce:
- 1 clove Garlic, pressed

- 1 cup Greek Yogurt

- kosher Salt, to taste

- juice from 1 Lemon

- 1 tbsp. fresh Dill

Directions:

1. Grease the Instant Pot with olive oil. Make a cut at the top of the bell peppers near the stem. Place feta cheese, onion, olives, tomatoes, cauliflower rice, salt, black pepper, garlic powder, and lemon juice into a bowl; mix well.

2. Fill up the bell peppers with the feta mixture and insert in the Instant Pot. Set on Manual and cook on High pressure for 20 minutes. When the timer beeps, allow the pressure to release naturally for 5 minutes, then do a quick pressure release.

3. To prepare the yogurt sauce, combine garlic, yogurt, lemon juice, salt, and fresh dill.

Nutrition: Calories 388, Protein 13.5g, Net Carbs 7.9g, Fat 32.4g

Shrimp with Linguine

Preparation Time: 10 minutes

Cooking Time: 10 minutes

Servings: 4

Ingredients:

- 1 lb. Shrimp, cleaned
- 1 lb. Linguine
- 1 tbsp. Butter
- ½ cup white Wine
- ½ cup Parmesan cheese, shredded
- 2 Garlic cloves, minced
- 1 cup Parsley, chopped
- Salt and Pepper, to taste
- ½ cup Coconut Cream, for garnish
- ½ Avocado, diced, for garnish
- 2 tbsp. fresh Dill, for garnish

Directions:

1. Melt the butter on Sauté. Stir in linguine, garlic cloves and parsley. Cook for 4 minutes

until aromatic. Add shrimp and white wine; season with salt and pepper, seal the lid.

2. Select Manual and cook for 5 minutes on High pressure. When ready, quick release the pressure. Unseal and remove the lid. Press Sauté, add the cheese and stir well until combined, for 30-40 seconds. Serve topped with the coconut cream, avocado, and dill.

Nutrition: Calories 412, Protein 48g, Net Carbs 5.6g, Fat 21g

Mexican Cod Fillets

Preparation Time: 10 minutes

Cooking Time: 10 minutes

Servings: 3

Ingredients:

- 3 Cod fillets
- 1 Onion, sliced
- 2 cups Cabbage
- Juice from 1 Lemon
- 1 Jalapeno Pepper
- ½ tsp Oregano
- ½ tsp Cumin powder
- ½ tsp Cayenne Pepper
- 2 tbsp. Olive oil
- Salt and black Pepper to taste

Directions:

1. Heat the oil on Sauté, and add onion, cabbage, lemon juice, jalapeño pepper, cayenne pepper, cumin powder and

oregano, and stir to combine. Cook for 8-10 minutes.

2. Season with salt and black pepper. Arrange the cod fillets in the sauce, using a spoon to cover each piece with some of the sauce. Seal the lid and press Manual. Cook for 5 minutes on High pressure. When ready, do a quick release and serve.

Nutrition: Calories 306, Protein 21g, Net Carbs 6.8g, Fat 19.4g

Simple Mushroom Chicken Mix

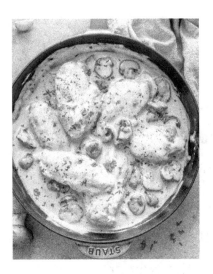

Preparation Time: 5 minutes

Cooking Time: 18 minutes

Servings: 2

Ingredients:

- 2 Tomatoes, chopped
- ½ lb. Chicken, cooked and mashed
- 1 cup Broccoli, chopped
- 1 tbsp. Butter
- 2 tbsp. Mayonnaise
- ½ cup Mushroom soup
- Salt and Pepper, to taste

- 1 Onion, sliced

Directions:

1. Once cooked, put the chicken into a bowl. In a separate bowl, mix the mayo, mushroom soup, tomatoes, onion, broccoli, and salt and pepper. Add the chicken.

2. Grease a round baking tray with butter. Put the mixture in a tray. Add 2 cups of water into the Instant Pot and place the trivet inside. Place the tray on top. Seal the lid, press Manual and cook for 14 minutes on High pressure. When ready, do a quick release.

Nutrition: Calories 561, Protein 28.5g, Net Carbs 6.3g, Fat 49.5g

Squash Spaghetti with Bolognese Sauce

Preparation Time: 5 minutes

Cooking Time: 10 minutes

Servings: 3

Ingredients:

- 1 large Squash, cut into 2 and seed pulp removed
- 2 cups Water
- Bolognese Sauce to serve

Directions:

1. Place the trivet and add the water. Add in the squash, seal the lid, select Manual and cook on High Pressure for 8 minutes. Once ready, quickly release the pressure. Carefully remove the squash; use two forks to shred the inner skin. Serve with Bolognese sauce.

Nutrition: Calories 37, Protein 0.9g, Net Carbs 7.8g, Fat 0.4g

Healthy Halibut Fillets

Preparation Time: 5 minutes

Cooking Time: 10 minutes

Servings: 2

Ingredients:

- 2 Halibut fillets
- 1 tbsp. Dill
- 1 tbsp. Onion powder
- 1 cup Parsley, chopped
- 2 tbsp. Paprika
- 1 tbsp. Garlic powder
- 1 tbsp. Lemon Pepper
- 2 tbsp. Lemon juice

Directions:

1. Mix lemon juice, lemon pepper, and garlic powder, and paprika, parsley, and dill and onion powder in a bowl. Pour the mixture in

the Instant pot and place the halibut fish

over it.

2. Seal the lid, press Manual mode and cook for

10 minutes on High pressure. When ready,

do a quick pressure release by setting the

valve to venting.

Nutrition: Calories 283, Protein 22.5g, Net Carbs

6.2g, Fat 16.4g

Clean Salmon with Soy Sauce

Preparation Time: 10 minutes

Cooking Time: 30 minutes

Servings: 2

Ingredients:

- 2 Salmon fillets
- 2 tbsp. Avocado oil
- 2 tbsp. Soy sauce
- 1 tbsp. Garlic powder
- 1 tbsp. fresh Dill to garnish
- Salt and Pepper, to taste

Directions:

1. To make the marinade, thoroughly mix the soy sauce, avocado oil, salt, pepper and garlic powder into a bowl. Dip salmon in the mixture and place in the refrigerator for 20 minutes.

2. Transfer the contents to the Instant pot. Seal, set on Manual and cook for 10 minutes

on high pressure. When ready, do a quick release. Serve topped with the fresh dill.

Nutrition: Calories 512, Protein 65g, Net Carbs 3.2g, Fat 21g

Simple Salmon with Eggs

Preparation Time: 2 minutes

Cooking Time: 5 minutes

Servings: 3

Ingredients:

- 1 lb. Salmon, cooked, mashed
- 2 Eggs, whisked
- 2 Onions, chopped
- 2 stalks celery, chopped
- 1 cup Parsley, chopped
- 1 tbsp. Olive oil
- Salt and Pepper, to taste

Directions:

1. Mix salmon, onion, celery, parsley, and salt and pepper, in a bowl. Form into 6 patties about 1 inch thick and dip them in the whisked eggs. Heat oil in the Instant pot on Sauté mode.

2. Add the patties to the pot and cook on both sides, for about 5 minutes and transfer to the plate. Allow to cool and serve.

Nutrition: Calories 331, Protein 38g, Net Carbs 5.3g, Fat 16g

Easy Shrimp

Preparation Time: 4 minutes

Cooking Time: 5 minutes

Servings: 2

Ingredients:

- 1 lb. Shrimp, peeled and deveined
- 2 Garlic cloves, crushed
- 1 tbsp. Butter.
- A pinch of red Pepper
- Salt and Pepper, to taste
- 1 cup Parsley, chopped

Directions:

1. Melt butter on Sauté mode. Add shrimp, garlic, red pepper, salt and pepper. Cook for 5 minutes, stirring occasionally the shrimp until pink. Serve topped with parsley.

Nutrition: Calories 245, Protein 45g, Net Carbs 4.8g, Fat 4g

Scallops with Mushroom Special

Preparation Time: 15 minutes

Cooking Time: 20 minutes

Servings: 2

Ingredients:

- 1 lb. Scallops
- 2 Onions, chopped
- 1 tbsp. Butter
- 2 tbsp. Olive oil
- 1 cup Mushrooms
- Salt and Pepper, to taste
- 1 tbsp. Lemon juice
- ½ cup Whipping Cream
- 1 tbsp. chopped fresh Parsley

Directions:

1. Heat the oil on Sauté. Add onions, butter, mushrooms, salt and pepper. Cook for 3 to 5 minutes. Add the lemon juice and scallops. Lock the lid and set to Manual mode.

2. Cook for 15 minutes on High pressure. When ready, do a quick pressure release and carefully open the lid. Top with a drizzle of cream and fresh parsley.

Nutrition: Calories 312, Protein 31g, Net Carbs 7.3g, Fat 10.4g

Delicious Creamy Crab Meat

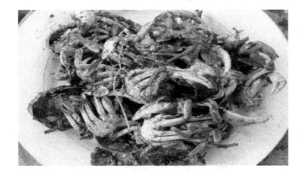

Preparation Time: 5 minutes

Cooking Time: 10 minutes

Servings: 3

Ingredients:

- 1 lb. Crab meat
- ½ cup Cream cheese
- 2 tbsp. Mayonnaise
- Salt and Pepper, to taste
- 1 tbsp. Lemon juice
- 1 cup Cheddar cheese, shredded

Directions:

1. Mix mayo, cream cheese, salt and pepper, and lemon juice in a bowl. Add in crab meat

and make small balls. Place the balls inside the pot. Seal the lid and press Manual.

2. Cook for 10 minutes on High pressure. When done, allow the pressure to release naturally for 10 minutes. Sprinkle the cheese over and serve!

Nutrition: Calories 443, Protein 41g, Net Carbs 2.5g, Fat 30.4g

Creamy Broccoli Stew

Preparation Time: 10 minutes

Cooking Time: 20 minutes

Servings: 4

Ingredients:

- 1 cup Heavy Cream
- 3 oz. Parmesan cheese
- 1 cup Broccoli florets
- 2 Carrots, sliced
- ½ tbsp. Garlic paste
- ¼ tbsp. Turmeric powder
- Salt and black Pepper, to taste
- ½ cup Vegetable broth
- 2 tbsp. Butter

Directions:

1. Melt butter on Sauté mode. Add garlic and sauté for 30 seconds. Add broccoli and carrots, and cook until soft, for 2-3 minutes. Season with salt and pepper.

2. Stir in the vegetable broth and seal the lid. Cook on Meat/Stew mode for 40 minutes. When ready, do a quick pressure release? Stir in the heavy cream.

Nutrition: Calories 239, Protein 8g, Net Carbs 5.1g, Fat 21.4g

Conclusion

The anti-inflammatory diet cookbook is the perfect resource for anyone who is suffering from inflammation. This cookbook has a special focus on reducing inflammation in the joints, cartilage, and muscles. Each recipe has been carefully developed to help reduce joint pain, joint stiffness, and even autoimmune disorders such as lupus and rheumatoid arthritis.

While most people associate food with comfort, a large number of foods are actually capable of having a dramatic impact on your health. Foods that are high in good fats (omega-3) are especially beneficial for many issues that affect the body. This cookbook provides recipes that are high in good fats and low in inflammatory foods like gluten and dairy. These recipes can be used to help create an anti-inflammatory diet that can help you feel better! The inflammatory disease will lead to many different health consequences and will even attack our most vital organs. The best way to do this is to prevent chronic inflammation in the first place. The next best thing is to recognize the signs and symptoms as early as possible, so proper interventions can be done to limit and reverse the impact of chronic inflammation. Inflammatory disease is the root cause of many long-term diseases, so ignoring the warning signs can create major consequences for your health.

Unfortunately, if the inflammatory disease gets out of control, preventative measures may be out of the question, and medical interventions will need to be done. Our goal is to prevent you from getting to this point. Lucky for us, many lifestyle changes can be performed to stop and reverse this disease process when it is still in its in advance stages. This is another reason why we should recognize and not ignore the signs and symptoms. A major lifestyle change we can commit to is a new diet plan. The anti-inflammatory diet is a meal plan that boasts healthy and nutritious cuisines, but still flavorful and appealing to the taste buds. There is a major myth out there that healthy food cannot be delicious. We have proven this myth wrong by providing numerous recipes from around the world that follow our healthy meal plan.

We hope that the information you read in this book gives you a better understanding of how the immune system functions and how a proper diet plan can help protect it and our other valuable cells and tissues. The recipes we have provided are just a starting point. Use them as a guide to create many of your dishes that follow the diet plan. Just make sure you use the proper ingredients and food groups. Also, for maximum results, follow the Anti-Inflammatory Diet food Guide Pyramid.

The next step is to take the instruction we have provided and begin taking steps to change your life and improve your health. Begin recognizing the signs and symptoms of chronic inflammation and make the necessary lifestyle changes to prevent further health problems. Start transitioning to the anti-inflammatory diet today by incorporating small meals into your schedule and increase the amount as tolerated. Within a short period, the diet will be a regular part of your routine. You will notice increased energy, improved mental function, a stronger and well-balanced immune system, reduction in chronic pain, some healthy weight loss, and overall better health outcomes. If you are ready to experience these changes, then wait no longer and begin putting your knowledge from this book into action.

CPSIA information can be obtained
at www.ICGtesting.com
Printed in the USA
BVHW092244260421
605885BV00002B/204